CRAVINGS
BOSS

The REAL Reason You Crave Food and a 5-Step Plan to Take Back Control

A practical guide on how to win the battle with your cravings for good.

NATALIA LEVEY, CNC

BALBOA.
PRESS
A DIVISION OF HAY HOUSE

Balboa Press books may be ordered through booksellers or by contacting:

Balboa Press
A Division of Hay House
1663 Liberty Drive
Bloomington, IN 47403
www.balboapress.com
1 (877) 407-4847

Print information available on the last page.

ISBN: 978-1-5043-4994-9 (sc)
ISBN: 978-1-5043-4996-3 (hc)
ISBN: 978-1-5043-4995-6 (e)

Library of Congress Control Number: 2016901775

Balboa Press rev. date: 03/10/2016

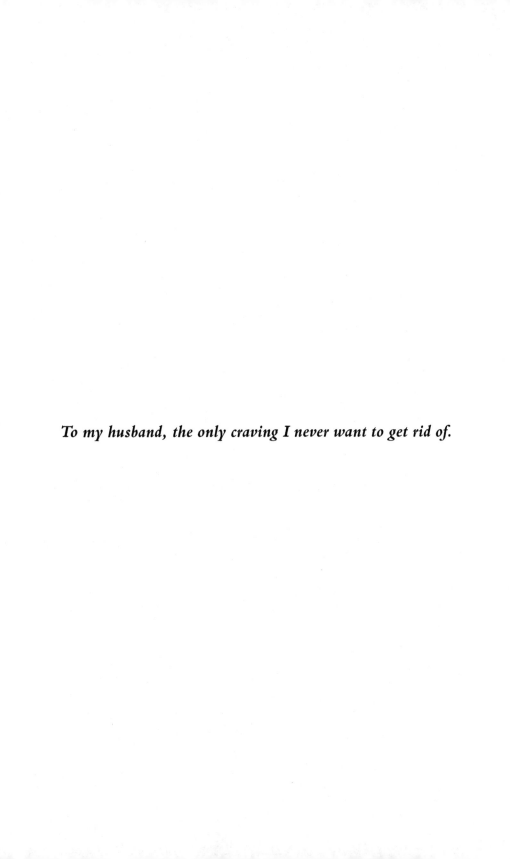

To my husband, the only craving I never want to get rid of.

CONTENTS

INTRODUCTION

If you are reading this book and you are anything like the millions of women who have struggled with diets, food and cravings, then you might be thinking, "I've tried it all—every diet, every program, every trick in the book, and yet I still find myself staring down the empty bucket of ice cream or into the vacant bag of chips as I realize that it was *me* who ate it all!"

Food cravings are like a cold—everyone is affected, and they can seem to come out of nowhere. But **the more you know how to be prepared, the less often you'll succumb to the lure of the chip bag.** I am about to arm you with superpowers that give you the ability to resist any food temptation thrown your way. That chocolate lava cake you usually cave in to? No thanks. The French fries that come with your sandwich? Not a chance. You are the boss of your cravings now, and I'll show you how.

I'm here to tell you that I've been there. I didn't always have it together. My cravings began during childhood. I grew up in Moscow, and about twice a year my family would stock up on 20 packages of kukuruznih palochek (sweet corn puffs), that were only available at certain times of the year. These special treats were supposed to last us six months, but without fail, the first five bags would be gone in just three days!

Cravings such as these become ingrained in us from an early age, but when we recognize the cause, we gain the upper hand. To this day, about twice a year I buy a bag, but now one bag lasts me a few days. Sometimes I glance lovingly at the bag in my pantry as a reminder of my past and my ability to exercise freedom of choice. And sometimes my choice is to eat them. The smell they make drives my husband crazy.

Imagine yourself at a lavish party, looking your best, meeting interesting people, and having the willpower to turn down the handsome stranger who urges you to eat the indulgences on his beautiful silver tray. I'm not asking you to turn down caviar and champagne—that's the Russian in me—but I *am* telling you that you can do this. Once you learn the REAL reasons why you crave food, you will have the confidence and motivation to make better choices. You may even discover a new hobby, like healthy cooking, growing your own food, or something totally non-food related.

Here is the thing: most nutrition and diet books merely present the facts. You get bogged down in details, and by the end of the book you have no energy left to actually implement the advice. I am not here to only teach you. I am here to empower you. I want you to take control of your cravings once and for all. I offer a different approach in this book. Your health is your business, and you are the boss. And when running a successful business, the best way to make a smart decision is to have all the information and facts in front of you. Do all the numbers add up? Do you need more resources? You can't act upon what you can't measure.

Before you run for the hills in fear of needing to multiply fractions just to get your cravings under control, rest assured that becoming a cravings boss is a piece of cake, er, a piece of salad. *Ahem.* You know what I mean. It also doesn't mean that you will deprive yourself. To the contrary, when you become more aware of the underlying causes and triggers of your cravings, they disappear. And once your cravings disappear, you will no longer need to deprive yourself because you won't be playing tug of war with your calories.

I wasn't always so health conscious. Although I grew up in a culture where cooking was a regular part of everyone's life, as I got older, and particularly after I moved to New York City, I became exposed to the culinary mecca. I began trying foods with difficult-to-pronounce names, and relying on prepared and convenient foods: hard to resist Chinese food delivered to my apartment ten minutes after hanging up the phone; hot dog vendors made famous by Hollywood blockbusters; endless bakeries . . .

Several years ago my curiosity about the inner workings of my body got the best of me. I plunged myself into the study of nutrition and the psychology of eating. While I had professional culinary training, it was more about combining flavours and cooking fundamentals. In the kitchen I always feel like an artist who gets to play with as many different media as possible—or one who can create a masterpiece using whatever is available that day. Sometimes that means coming up with something delicious using only three or four ingredients. I get so inspired by trips to local fresh markets during my travels, at home, farms, or restaurants in tiny Italian villages, as well as by other amazing chefs. Nature has become my muse.

My understanding of the beautiful complexity of the human body (and how to fuel it for optimum performance) came later. Becoming a certified health coach and nutritional consultant was a natural step for me in personal growth. Now I get to work with so many interesting people and help them become their own artists, doctors, investigators, nurses, and chefs. When it comes to making health decisions, you have to utilize all of the above traits.

My true first love is cooking (my hubby will argue this!), I now get to blend that love with the knowledge I gained through my Health Coach training from the Institute for Integrative Nutrition. Ultimately, I went on to become a Certified Nutritional Consultant by The American Association of Nutritional Consultants.

During my studies I learned about so many dietary theories. Aside from having strange and unsavoury names, some of these diets have unrealistic guidelines of what you should eat. To my surprise, some don't take into consideration personal, biochemical, environmental, and other variables.

What I took away from these many theories is that there is no one diet for everyone. You may be a Paleo gal. Or maybe vegetarianism is your thing. Perhaps you need to avoid gluten or dairy. You won't hear me preaching about how you need to eat. It's not my style. Instead, I want to get to know you. And most of all, I want you to get to know yourself. That's what this book is about. I want you to discover the messages your body is trying to send you. You interpret them as cravings, but when you dig below the surface, you will find that your body is sharing its wisdom. Now it's time to listen. I'll show you how.

With my combined culinary skills and deepened understanding of nutrition, I founded Healthy Intent, a lifestyle brand that helps entrepreneurs to incorporate BOSS {beyond ordinary self-care strategies} plan into their lives, so they can become more productive and reach their health and wellness goals through focused education, worksheets, and inspiration. This book is one of my efforts to help you better understand your body, your food and how to be well.

Now, let's can those cravings, shall we boss?

TERMINATION LETTER TO SELF-SABOTAGE

Have you been in a pattern of devouring health advice and going in full force only to crash and burn, back where you started or worse? I know the feeling. Once we look at the amazing cards in our hands, we go all in. We dive off the cliff of uncertainty and pick up speed as we implement positive changes. But eventually we fall. Hard.

Nope. Not this time. You are about to be armed with powerful tools and strategies that will prevent you from playing tug-of-war with your cravings. You can become the unstoppable force, the capable-of-anything-I-set-my-mind-to rockstar superhero you envision yourself to be.

It's time to say goodbye to self-sabotage. You are about to implement your new business plan. Take out your favorite colored pen and a piece of paper (pink works)—it's time to write the termination letter, boss.

Dearest Self-Sabotage,

It has come to my attention that your contributions to my life have inhibited my personal growth potential. Your efforts to disrupt and distract me from reaching my annual goals are no longer needed. You have worthlessly served me for [insert age] years. In fact, I've taken personal pay cuts in order to continually allocate funds that only benefitted your expanding power.

I no longer need your services. Your position has been terminated, effective immediately.
Your spot has been filled by a new, awesome force called Self-Respect.
I understand that being replaced by a super-intelligent awesomeness is going to totally crush you, and I am prepared to deal with your scheming ways to crawl back in. Take comfort in the knowledge that you, too, have great transformation potential.
I encourage you to sign up for the training sessions with Self-Respect.
All my best.

No longer yours truly,
[insert your name here]

POTENTIAL DANGERS
OF OVEREATING

When I was pregnant and lived in New York City, the guy behind the counter at Häagen Dazs ice cream shop knew not only my name, but also my order. Weekly trips to that little corner shop led me to gain extra weight in my last trimester, and my doctor, beloved Jacques Moritz, threatened me with the possibility of gestational diabetes. Fortunately, my daughter was born a healthy 9 lbs 4 oz, and I quickly forgot about the threat of diabetes and carried on with my life. But I continued to indulge myself for years without thinking. I wish I had known then everything I know now.

The fact is, most of the time cravings lead to overeating. In fact, physical cravings- those that are triggered by imbalances in the body's physiology- often lead to serious food addictions.

According to the Food Addiction Institute, "There is now more scientific verification for physical craving as a part of food addiction than there was for physical craving with regard to alcoholism and other drug addictions when they were first designated as substance use disorders."[1]

Wouldn't it be great (and ultimately cheaper and healthier) if we instead had cravings for exercise, vegetables, or even drawing mandalas or watching squirrels? Once our bodies are reset and cleansed from candida, unhealthy gut bacteria, inflammation, it is possible to start having healthy cravings for green smoothies or certain vegetables or fruit.

The topic of food addictions still causes a lot of controversy among scientists, and the information presented in chapter "THE MANY CAUSES OF CRAVINGS and HOW TO DEAL WITH THEM" has been compiled from my research and observations. What I have learned is that each person's experience is truly individual and is based on factors such as age, gender, and individual biochemistry, among others.

Scientists have established that overeating can lead to obesity, diabetes, high blood pressure, elevated cholesterol, fatty liver, heart disease, and many more serious conditions. That includes spending too much money on a larger-sized wardrobe and the pain of knowing that you're wearing your fat jeans, or something glamorously baggy. "Oversized sweaters are in, haven't you heard?"

Just like medications come with side effects and warning labels, so should food packages and commercials. Instead of the usual warnings in commercials, "If you are concerned about your ability to perform in the bedroom, talk to your doctor about [insert impotence medication here]. You may experience headache, stomach upset, back pain, dizziness, or an erection that lasts for days, etc.," why not a warning on food packaging and advertisements? "Consuming one serving of cookies may lead to impulsive feelings that cause you to devour the entire package at night when your family thinks you're in bed sleeping, leading to high blood sugar, diabetes, and possibly cardiovascular disease. Consult with your doctor before eating these cookies to determine whether you might be at risk."

Many functional medicine doctors today believe that food is medicine. Functional medicine addresses the underlying causes of disease, using a systems-oriented approach and engaging both patient and practitioner in a therapeutic partnership. This form of integrative medicine is poised to change the way medicine is practiced. But most of us weren't raised to believe that food is medicine. How were you raised to think about food?

Food is just food. It keeps hunger at bay and brings families and friends together at the dinner table. Sometimes it comforts us after a stressful day, or maybe helps us get over a painful breakup. You've seen the all-too-familiar movie scene: "He broke up with me," says the woman while sitting in her living room in pajamas at three in the afternoon eating ice cream out of the carton, the room an explosion of pizza delivery boxes and tissues. This is hardly food as medicine.

While manufacturers spend millions of dollars creating foods that continually make us crave more and coming up with clever marketing campaigns to keep selling so-called "energy" foods, we are left to deal with our addictions and health consequences. Some commercials make foods look so good that you end up eating three bars in a row, only to crash an hour later.

Years ago I thought I had perfected my method of dealing with cravings: talk to myself sternly, make empty promises to not do it again, spend thirty extra minutes on the treadmill, work a lot from home, or not work at all, avoid seeing friends or putting on a bathing suit, and when all else fails, shop for larger sized clothes! It didn't occur to me back then to look at exactly what my cravings were or why they were happening.

This book contains a great deal of wisdom that I have accumulated over the years and have learned through my clients' and my own personal experiences. I am sharing this information with you because I wish I had learned it sooner. Some of the solutions are unconventional, but I promise it will be a fun experiment.

5-STEP PLAN TO TAKE
BACK CONTROL

I hear so many marketing slogans: "Invest in your college education," "Invest in your retirement," "Invest in your future." What about investing in your health? Frankly, if you don't take care of your health, your college, adult, and golden years will be pretty lousy.

Think back to the last time you made a decision with misplaced conviction. "Yes, these shoes *must* become a part of my collection." Or "No, I'm too sick to go out. It's definitely the flu." Only too soon you realize that you don't have money for the heels or you're suddenly feeling better and can go out to that concert.

I know there have been many times that I've said yes to something but didn't really mean it. And those events, conversations, interactions, and visits made me feel miserable.

It's time to conjure up authentic conviction—the conviction that gets you out of bed every morning at 6 a.m. to face your day; the conviction that led you to exchange vows with your spouse; and the conviction that will keep you reading about how to be the boss of your cravings throughout this book.

This conviction that we all possess is what I'm calling out to right now. But it requires work. Come on, it's time to start flexing your muscles. I've got an exercise program for your conviction.

1. **Be strong in your convictions.** Sound confident when you say YES or NO to daily temptations. Say it like you mean it.
2. **Be flexible.** Understand that there will be times to bend the rules. Trees and buildings are designed to be flexible so they don't break in the wind. Your eating habits need to be flexible on occasion.
3. **Find endurance.** You are in it for the long haul. This is not a quick-fix diet. It's a lifestyle change that you take with you wherever you go. The rest of your life starts now.

Time is of the essence. The following plan will help you implement what you've learned and save you the time and suffering of giving in to your health-sabotaging cravings.

When you feel a craving come on, follow this 5-step plan. Let's call it "Cravings Operating Agreement."

1. **Pause. Have a two-minute board meeting with yourself.**

   When you take a moment to pause, take in your surroundings, and notice what is going on in your body and mind, you will be better equipped to understand and deal with your craving. Mindless surrender to your cravings is a sure way to end up at the bottom of your snack pile, sticky and guilt-ridden. Take pause. Set your timer for two minutes. You need it to assess the situation. Once you take that first bite, it's all over and much harder to stop.

2. **Examine the facts.**

   As you will learn in this book, there are fifteen different causes of cravings. Consider the possible reasons for your craving so that you can move forward appropriately. Once you've narrowed it down, flip back to the corresponding section and read about what solutions you can implement immediately or over time.

3. **Pinpoint the trigger.**

   The trigger of your cravings is the moment when the specific cause of your cravings comes into play. You are triggered by these underlying factors—and they're everywhere. Once you understand the causes of your

9

cravings, you will be able to recognize when they are triggered.

4. **Promote your imagination.**

Visualizing your potential outcome will rewire your initial brain response. Imagine yourself at your healthiest—able to turn down cravings and choose the foods that fuel your body and mind. Imagine that you are already in control. See it happen as though it were already real. There's a super fun exercise corresponding with this section. Keep on reading.

5. **Fire those cravings.**

Having an understanding of why your craving exists and what triggered it will help you take appropriate action steps. Worksheets at the end of this book will provide you with data and tools for creating a new strategy for success, leaving your cravings behind.

STEP 1. PAUSE

Have you ever sent or received a text message without first thinking it through? Have you ever made a decision without weighing all the pros and cons or having a clear picture in front of you?

Here is what happens when you make rushed decisions:

1. **You feel regret.** Acting before thinking is a sure way to put the proverbial foot in your mouth—or cake in your mouth, as the case may be.
2. **You avoid taking responsibility for your bad decision.** You launch into defense mode, trying to cover for your slip up. "I can just work this off at the gym, no problem." Overtime doesn't always pay double.

3. **You experience loss of investment (i.e. waistline).** When I talk about investment, I mean your health investment—all the good nutrition and self-care practices that you undertake.

4. **You waste valuable resources**. All the work you put in—your time, money, health and energy to "run the business"—is squandered when you make decisions without thinking them through.

Take a two-minute time-out to assess the facts and bring down the intensity of your urge. Allow yourself to take three deep breaths. Grab a glass of water. Taking this moment for yourself will put you in charge of your impulse to eat something you'll regret 10 minutes later, or next day while trying to get into the skinny jeans before a party, or a week later while packing for a beach getaway.

Taking this pause will help you to be more mindful—more aware of what is going on in your immediate environment—body and mind—right here, right now. Mindfulness can be your new personal assistant. When you need an objective perspective and help in identifying the best strategy for successful outcome, mindfulness is by your side and at your service.

By practicing silence towards your cravings, you may even intimidate them into crawling right back into the box from which they have appeared. Then you'll be able to clarify your intentions, review all the possible outcomes and plot a new course.

STEP 2. EXAMINE THE FACTS

What is a craving?

A craving is an uncontrollable desire, in this case, to consume a specific food.

Cravings are powerful messages that your body sends to inform you about an underlying imbalance. Think of it as your internal snail mail system. Your goal is to learn to decode these messages and respond appropriately.

Cravings can sometimes be subtle, like ripples on the lake from a slight breeze; other times they might hit you like a ton a bricks. Must. Have. Pizza. Subtle cravings are fairly easy to manage. Strong cravings, on the other hand, can get ugly—reach for one too many snack cakes and you'll be left with devastating feelings of guilt, a puffy face, a bloated abdomen, pants that don't fit, and bruised confidence. It's likely that you have dealt with both types of cravings. But now it's time to tell them who's boss.

Cravings can be loosely categorized as emotional, physiological or environmental. An emotional craving comes on when certain emotions are felt, like sadness or anxiety. A physiological, or physical, craving arises when the body is in need of a certain nutrient or when the brain receives certain signals. An environmental craving is induced when you find yourself amidst the tantalizing smell of pizza or when all your friends are sharing cheesecake smothered in clouds of whipped cream at dinner.

Cravings often tag along with the all-too-familiar emotion, guilt. How many times have you thrown up your hands, pleading, "What's wrong with me?!" That's your old frenemy, guilt. It sends you straight to the gym where you sign a year's contract and attend every Buns Burner class for a month, only to fizzle out when some bon-bons from a corner bakery win the debate between working out or working on your sweet tooth. The cravings-and-guilt cycle is vicious.

Don't get me wrong, signing up for a gym membership is a great idea. In fact, I'm an avid gym goer. I've been working out with a trainer consistently for seven years now. It's a big part of my life. But if you continue to give in to your cravings because you don't understand what they are really telling you, then your gym membership is a waste of money.

Trips to the gym should not be used as an excuse to consume more calories or indulge. If you are working out to earn that cupcake (or three cupcakes, or an extra glass of wine with an accidental block of cheese, ahem), then you're in for disappointment.

One of my absolute favorite quotes is "Abs are made in the kitchen." (On the other hand, so are potbellies, spare tires and love handles.)

Just picture different foods dressed up as people, in their Sunday best, trying to find ways to make themselves look most appetizing. Which foods in your kitchen, at your favorite restaurant or takeout joint would have the loudest voice? When you find yourself falling for the allure of your strongest craving food, picture it screaming at you just like that annoying stranger, relative or coworker who always tries to be the center of attention. It's time to limit your interaction with craving foods, if not get rid of them altogether.

Now envision some of the healthiest and most nutritious foods. They are humble and polite, just waiting to be discovered by you. They have big dreams, and are excited to start making a huge impact on your world, but they do so under the radar. Just like people, sometimes the quiet voices will surprise you the most. That piece of broccoli is gently waiving its pretty green head at you, saying, "Hey there. I'm waiting for you here with my friends, cauliflower and carrots. We'd love to make a delivery of our best nutrients to your cells. Wait. Don't walk away . . . Please. We just want to be loved."

After my workouts, I am often absolutely starving. I have learned to listen to the messages of my cravings, and I now choose a healthy option that helps my muscles recover. In the old days, when my cravings controlled me, I would eat a piece of candy to "reward" myself for burning tons of calories. Those days are over. Now I go for a veggie protein smoothie instead.

Cravings still hit me at different times of day, often at night when I have a few minutes to finally relax. Before I learned to be the boss of my cravings, I could end up packing in over 1,000 calories in empty snacks just before bedtime. Sound familiar? Now I make a relaxing cup of tea, and it usually satisfies me. But I first go through the 5-step process explained at the beginning of this book.

You, too will be the boss of your cravings after reading this book and implementing the solutions.

What is the difference between cravings and hunger?

There are quite a few significant differences between cravings and hunger.

You have surely experienced that critical moment after not eating for a few hours—that moment when you are capable of eating anything and everything put in front of you. I'm not a big fan of cheese, but if I've gone many hours without a proper meal, cheese is suddenly delicious. I am particularly susceptible to cheese during travel.

I remember talking to my grandmother about her experiences during World War II. There was no food available, so they would eat patties made out of grass. That's true hunger. If you read any history books about people who have suffered during times of crisis, the descriptions of real hunger will bring tears to your eyes.

We don't even have to look far; hunger is still a very real problem all over the world—even in highly developed countries. In fact, many kids are only able to eat because schools provide free breakfasts and lunches.

I often think about the discipline it takes for people to function and stay positive during such difficult times. It makes me reevaluate the way I look and think about food. For many of those people food is necessary for basic survival. It makes a triple-decker fudge sundae seem that much more extravagant.

The table below shows main differentiating factors between cravings and hunger. Consider these differences the next time you reach out for something to eat. Ask yourself, "When was the last time I ate?" "Am I truly hungry or is this a craving?" If it's hunger that drives your desire for food, take notice of the fact that you are likely to overcompensate by eating more than you need. As they say, "Your eyes are bigger than your stomach." Portion control is a must!

If you're hungry and yet you've eaten in the past couple hours, you're likely being lured by a craving. Keep reading to learn about what you can do to curb those cravings. Remember, you're the boss. It's time to fire your cravings.

CRAVINGS	HUNGER
Usually associated with guilt	A biological need of the body
Involve mental negotiations with yourself	Not focused on a specific food
Often involve comfort foods	Can be satisfied with an available meal
Triggered by an underlying cause	Doesn't pass until satisfied
Will pass with time or management techniques	Accompanied by major physical discomfort

TYPES OF FOOD CRAVINGS

Foods you consume or crave vary in taste, texture and temperature.

Your body is able to recognize five different tastes: sweet, sour, bitter, salty and umami (savory). You likely gravitate towards some tastes more than others. Think about the texture of foods you are most attracted to. Something that melts in your mouth or something crunchy? Now consider the effect that temperature has on your food preferences. Maybe you prefer your foods piping hot or like to drink beverages that are ice cold.

The taste, texture and temperature of your foods can strongly affect what foods you crave. What if you knew that food scientists are being paid a lot of money to create foods that are so addictive that it becomes physically impossible to resist taking another bite? Make no mistake, that package of pastries is calling your name because it's manufactured to do so.

Scary thought, I know. Don't get mad and start making a list of someone to blame. People are just doing their jobs really well. How well are you going to do yours?

Let's take a look at two major food cravings: salt and sugar.

Salt

For centuries, salt has been recognized not only as a currency and a food preservative, but also for its medicinal use. Over the past few decades, salt has gotten a bad rap for its role in raising blood pressure, but there is currently a lot of controversy regarding the subject. As it turns out, too much salt as well as too little salt can be detrimental to health, so recommendations to reduce salt intake must consider what the intake is to begin with.[2] After reviewing a significant amount of research, I conclude that there are many other factors that contribute to the rise in blood pressure, including raised BMI, sodium sensitivity, genetics, age and chronic dehydration.[3] It is important to keep in mind that it usually takes a combination of factors over time to wreak havoc on our health.

Sodium is necessary for preventing dehydration, regulating fluid balance of the body, proper transmission of nerve impulses and for normal functioning of cells.

According to the FDA, the words *salt* and *sodium* are not synonymous, but they are often used interchangeably. Salt, also known by its chemical name sodium chloride, is a crystal-like compound that is abundant in nature and used to flavor and preserve food. Sodium is one of the two chemical elements found in salt.

According to one study, "Commonly occurring events that cause mild fluid loss and electrolyte imbalance in infancy, as well as prenatally, predict the avidity for salt in adolescents." In other words, once sodium deficiency is experienced, salt cravings can persist later in life.[4]

Fereydoon Batmanghelidj, MD, an internationally renowned doctor, researcher, author and advocate of the natural healing power of water, recommends ingesting small amounts of salt with water as part of his Water Cure program.[5]

From my own personal experience, I have discovered that placing a small grain of Himalayan pink salt on the tip of my tongue stopped feelings of nausea. (This makes sense when you consider that our bodies lose significant amounts of sodium during vomiting and diarrhea.) I concluded that *salt craving is an indicator of a sodium deficiency*, a theory that has been confirmed by research.[6]

According to Paul Pitchford, author of *Healing with Whole Foods*, "In Chinese physiology . . . desire for salt may reflect an internal wish for a more emotionally safe foundation." He states, "A craving for salt is perhaps a craving not only for the many minerals normally associated with unrefined salt but for some of the same minerals that are lacking in commercially grown food."

While there are many different types of salts available, those derived from the Earth's minerals present a much more nutritious choice than common table salt, which lack minerals. Including moderate amounts of such salts in your meals will help ensure that you receive the benefits of salts. Natural wholesome foods are low in sodium, so adding a bit of salt when eating such foods will only enhance flavor and nutrient intake. Beware of processed foods, however, which usually contain very high amounts of salt, making your kidneys work overtime.

Hidden sources of salt:

- Anything cured or in a brine
- Baked goods
- Canned goods
- Condiments
- Deli meats
- Fast food
- Processed cheese

STRATEGIES FOR DEALING WITH SALT CRAVINGS

- **Avoid processed foods.** Processed food products are notoriously high in sodium, which is used as a flavor enhancer, preservative and to improve texture. According to the FDA, 77 percent of American's sodium intake in 2012 was from packaged and restaurant food.
- **Read labels.** According to food labeling laws, products labeled as "sodium free" or "salt free" cannot exceed 5 mg of sodium per serving. A product with a "low

sodium" claim must not exceed 140 mg per serving. A "no salt added" or "unsalted" claim on the label does not mean the food is sodium free.

- **Use whole, unrefined salt and explore other spices.** Basil is great to use in soups and salads, and on vegetables, fish and meats. Cayenne pepper is tasty on meats and poultry, and in stews and sauces. Cilantro pairs well with meats, sauces, stews and rice. Ground mustard on beef, chicken, lamb, pork and cheese is divine. Rosemary is best used in salads and on vegetables, fish and meats. Another great spice, turmeric is wonderful on chicken, fish or beef.

- **Keep your stress levels under control.** Your adrenal glands are in charge of releasing the hormone cortisol in response to stress and the hormone aldosterone, which is responsible for regulating the level of salt and fluid in your blood. Chronic stress causes your adrenal glands to burn out, lowering their production of hormones. The kidneys will try to even out the balance by excreting salt, causing your body to crave it more. Incorporating daily meditation practice, relaxation techniques and working with alternative medicine practitioners have yielded great results for stress relief.

- **Drink ample amounts of water.** Adequate water intake will prevent dehydration, which triggers cravings that you might misinterpret as a need for food.

- **Try snacking on kelp chips.** Kelp is a great source of many natural sea minerals.
- **Select frozen vegetables instead of canned.** Frozen vegetables typically don't have added salt. If you do use canned, rinse them under cold water first.
- **Add salt only at the end of the cooking process.** This way you minimize the chances of over-saturating the food with salt.

If you are interested in reading more, I recommend the following resources:

1. *Salt: A World History* by Mark Kurlansky
2. Morris MJ, et al., "Salt craving: The psychobiology of pathogenic sodium intake." *Physiol Behav.* 2008 Aug 6; 94(5): 709–721. http://www.ncbi.nlm.nih.gov/pmc/articles/PMC2491403/#R1
3. Stamler R., "Implications of the INTERSALT study." *Hypertension.* 1991;17 (Suppl1):I16–I20. http://hyper.ahajournals.org/content/17/1_Suppl/I16.full.pdf

Sugar

Sugar is found in almost every processed food on the market today. It is used as a flavor enhancer more often than any other seasoning, including salt. I can almost guarantee that if you grab an inexpensive processed food from your local grocer, it will be loaded with sugar. Manufacturers are well aware of sugar's addictive quality.

People who are caught in this addictive loop usually drink several sugary sodas per day or consume large quantities of candy, processed sweets or packaged, ready-to-eat goodies. If you recognize yourself in these words, you're not alone.

Did you know the average American eats 152 pounds of sugar per year? One hundred and fifty two pounds. POUNDS! A baby giraffe weighs that much! That's approximately twenty-two teaspoons per day and it only takes about two cans of soda to reach this daily maximum. According to a paper by researcher Serge H. Ahmed, PhD, **sugar has been found to be eight times as addictive as cocaine.**[7] If that statistic doesn't scare the crap out of you, I don't know what will.

Sugar triggers constant cravings and weight gain due to the release of hormones in the liver and because it upsets the carbohydrate/protein balance. Mark Hyman, MD, author of *The Blood Sugar Solution 10-Day Detox Diet* and Director of The Cleveland Clinic Center for Functional Medicine, says, "First, your body becomes insulin resistant, and therefore you have to pump out more insulin in an attempt to keep your blood sugar normal. Insulin is a powerful fat-storage hormone, one that encourages your body to pack on dangerous belly fat. High levels of insulin produced through all the sugar and fructose consumption block the leptin signals in your brain, so your body thinks it is starving even after a Big Mac, fries and a large soda."

If you think that you can solve your sugar cravings by switching to artificial sweeteners, think again. According to Frank Lipman, MD, an internationally recognized expert in the fields of integrative and functional medicine, artificial sweeteners do not prevent weight gain.

If you're using artificial sweeteners to maintain or lose weight, you're probably doing more harm than good. Those little pastel color packages give the illusion of healthy, low-calorie alternatives, but there is little legitimate research to support their benefits.

Some alarming studies conclude that artificial sweeteners also *trigger cravings by tricking your brain into thinking it will actually get sugar.* These super-sweeteners flood your taste buds with overly sweet stimulus, which pushes your sweetness threshold even higher. Even if you do not crave real sugar, these artificial sweeteners interfere with the release of satiety hormones. By the time your body signals catch up, you're already craving more.

Certain artificial sweeteners kill good gut bacteria, which can leave you feeling bloated, nauseous, unsatisfied and just plain icky, simply put. These toxic little packages are full of negative side effects that are zapping your health.

In fact, a recent study revealed that heating sucralose—think about those yellow packets added to your hot coffee—creates a chemical compound similar to dioxin, a known carcinogen.[8] Yikes! Aspartame has been shown to cause cancer in lab rats and kill off significant amounts of those essential good gut bacteria. For years, saccharine has carried a warning label boldly declaring: "Use of this product may be hazardous to your health." Double yikes!

Add other side effects such as rashes, migraines, gas, bloating, dizziness, cramps and diarrhea, and you'll wonder what these products are doing on your grocery shelves.

While it is true that you need adequate supplies of dietary carbohydrates to create the glucose (sugar) that your body needs to energize itself, overeating foods high in simple carbohydrates causes too much sugar to be released into your blood. When this happens, your body produces extra insulin.

The more insulin that is released into your bloodstream, the more resistant your cells become to its action. When cells become insulin resistant, unable to shuffle sugar from your blood into cells, your blood sugar will rise. When there is too much sugar in the blood, it gets processed into fat by the liver and stored away—in your saddlebags.

Insulin is one of the main fat storage hormones. While insulin is shuffling sugar out of the blood, the decrease in blood sugar triggers a release of other chemicals in the body whose purpose is to raise blood sugar, most prominently adrenaline, which can cause jitters, a racing heart or over emotional reactions to common stimuli. This is yet one more reason to watch what types of sugars you eat, how much, and at what time of day!

How to spot sugar on food labels:

One of the easiest ways to recognize sugar on a food label is by identifying the -ose suffix. When you find words that end in -ose, there's a good chance it is sugar.

Names for added sugars		
Used in foods and beverages		
1. Agave nectar	18. Demerara sugar	35. Lactose
2. Anhydrous dextrose	19. Crystalline fructose	36. Maltose
3. Barley malt	20. Diatase	37. Maple syrup
4. Beet sugar	21. Date sugar	38. Molasses
5. Blackstrap molasses	22. Dehydrated fruit juice	39. Palm sugar
6. Brown sugar	23.. Dextrin	40. Pancake syrup
7. Brown rice syrup	24. Dextrose	41. Raw sugar
8. Cane sugar	25. Evaporated cane juice	42. Rice syrup
9. Cane juice	26. Fructose (high fructose corn syrup)	43. Refiners syrup
10. Caramel	27. Fruit juice concentrate	44. Saccharose
11. Carob syrup	28. Galactose	45. Sucrose
12. Coconut sugar	29. Glucomalt	46. Sugar
13. Coconut palm sugar	30. Glucose	47. Turbinado sugar
14. Confectioner's sugar	31. Grape juice concentrate	48. White sugar
15. Corn sweetener	32. Grape sugar	49. Xylose
16. Corn syrup	33. Honey	50. Yellow sugar
17.Crystal dextrose	34. Invert sugar	

There are six FDA-approved food additives in the United States that function as **high-intensity sweeteners:** saccharin, aspartame, acesulfame potassium (Ace-K), sucralose, neotame, and advantame. They are considered high-intensity sweeteners because they are many times sweeter than table sugar.

Glycemic index is a measure of the effect certain foods have on blood sugar levels. The lower a food's glycemic index or glycemic load, the less it affects blood sugar and thus, insulin levels.

Watermelon, pineapple and bananas have the highest glycemic index, while grapefruit, apples and pears have some of the lowest. The riper the fruit, the sweeter it is. High-fiber fruits and vegetables are best because fiber helps lower the absorption rate of sugar into the bloodstream.

Now that you know why sugar has such a huge effect on how you feel and how your body operates, it's time to get your sugar cravings in check, boss.

STRATEGIES TO GET SUGAR CRAVINGS UNDER CONTROL

- **Reduce or eliminate caffeine.** Caffeine creates a roller coaster of ups and downs including blood sugar swings and dehydration. This can cause you to crave something sweet to level you off. Save the roller coaster ride for the amusement park.
- **Drink water.** Sweet cravings can be a sign of dehydration. Reach for water or organic green tea before soda. Have fun and add some fresh fruit and herbs to your water to make it a refreshing spa experience.

MAKE YOUR OWN SPA WATER
Watermelon + Rosemary
Grapefruit + Basil
Cucumber + Strawberry + Mint
Lemon + Lime + Orange
Pineapple + Mango
Blackberry + Honeydew
Raspberry + Goji Berry
Lavender + Vanilla
Rosehip + Black Currant
Apple + Kiwi + Pear

- **Eat sweet vegetables and fruit.** They are naturally sweet, healthy and delicious. The more you eat natural sugars, the less you will crave the white stuff.

- **Avoid chemical or artificial sweeteners.** Stick to the natural stuff like maple syrup, brown rice syrup, agave, dried fruit, stevia and barley malt. Consider growing an actual stevia plant as a fun gardening project.

- **Get physically active.** Simple activities like walking or yoga can help curb sugar cravings. An active lifestyle helps to balance blood sugar levels, boost energy and reduce tension.

- **Get more sleep, rest and relaxation.** When overtired or stressed, you are more likely to reach for something sweet because it's a quick energy boost. Stay well rested and you won't be tempted.

- **Evaluate the amount of animal food you eat.**
  According to yin-yang principles of eating (macrobiotics
  and traditional Chinese medicine, for example), eating
  too much animal food (yang) can lead to cravings for
  sweets (yin). For some individuals, imbalances can also
  occur with too *little* animal protein. Find a balance that
  works for you.

- **Eliminate fat-free or low-fat packaged snack
  foods.** These foods contain high quantities of sugar to
  compensate for lack of flavor and fat. Don't be fooled.

- **Experiment with spices.** Coriander, cinnamon,
  nutmeg, cloves and cardamom are tantalizing flavors
  that will naturally sweeten your foods and thus reduce
  cravings.

- **Find sweetness in non-food ways!** Not every craving
  is a signal that your body biologically requires sugar.
  Cravings often have a psychological component. You
  may just need a little more love in your life. Hug your
  friend, lover, pet or family member. Take a look at your
  relationships. You may fill your craving simply by filling
  up on love.

- **Talk to your doctor about adding an L-glutamine
  supplement.** Glutamine is an amino acid that plays an
  important role in balancing blood sugar levels.

Sugar cravings be gone SMOOTHIE

This smoothie has no added sugars—only a combination of natural flavors to delight your taste buds. It's my favorite.

Ingredients:

1 cup ice

8 oz. coconut water (or goji berry infused green tea)

½ cup mixed greens. Whatever you have on hand: kale, spinach, arugula, dandelion greens, chard)

1 green apple

¼ cup chopped cucumber

3-4 mint leaves

2-3 sprigs of parsley

2-3 basil leaves

Juice of ¼ lime

1 Tablespoon almond butter

Optional: 1 scoop of organic plant protein

Method:

Blend well in the high-speed blender.

Keep in mind that the consistency of this drink will be juice-like, but with all the benefits of fiber.

To "ease" yourself into drinking this beautiful savory drink, you may start with adding ¼ cup of pineapple or watermelon to the mix, gradually reducing the amount.

An apple can be substituted with 1 pear or ½ cup of blueberries.

THE MANY CAUSES OF CRAVINGS AND HOW TO DEAL WITH THEM

1. Emotional imbalances

Unsatisfying relationships, stressful jobs, disappointing sex life and emotional highs and lows can all cause excessive binging or deprivation eating. Remember the break-up movie scene? When emotions run high, the body sends craving cues in order to obtain "rewards" from the brain, even if temporary. It's always best to seek out non-food related rewards first. There is whole chapter later on about changing your reward system.

When was the first time you bought a ticket for the emotional rollercoaster? Are you still on that ride? Or do you receive a monthly subscription of emotions, gradually increasing over time? Let's take a look at how this might play out.

Fear. Fear and worry show up throughout the day. You may be nervously anticipating your next meeting, worried about a conversation you had, or simply anxious about how to get everything done on your to-do list.

Sadness. We all experience sadness at certain points in our lives. Some people experience deeper sadness and for longer periods of time. You may find yourself turning to food to fill an emotional void, as though the solution to your problems can be found at the bottom of an ice cream pint.

Anger. Anger tends to swoop in before we even realize what happened, stealing the show and leaving everyone feeling worse in the end. To bury the shame and guilt that comes afterward, food often becomes a main focus. You may have noticed that you turn to food after coming down from an angry altercation.

Fortunately, you can address emotional imbalances in many ways that do not involve food.

A good boss knows the importance of personal time—and allows her employees to take it! To be prepared for emotional disruptions in your life, develop a list of self-care practices that you can implement when the need arises. The specific practices will vary from person to person. For one person, self-care might take the form of a long walk in nature, while for another person it might include a hot bath and a cup of tea.

Some self-care, however, is virtually universal. Soothing music works as a form of relaxation for almost anyone because the heart begins to automatically lower to match the beats per minute of the music. Similarly, meditation and deep breathing are well documented to provide relaxation benefits in the short term, and a wide array of mental and emotional benefits when practiced long term.

It might take time and experimentation to find the right combination of self-care practices that work to relax and reward you emotionally so that you don't give in to your food cravings and eat food that isn't good for you. The amount of time you invest in finding a non-food solution to emotional disruptions is time well spent, as it will allow you to address your emotional issues in a healthy, balanced way. If one self-care practice doesn't work, resist the urge to solve your problems by giving into cravings and try another until you begin to feel better. The sooner you find a way to handle your upsets without food, the better off you will be.

Keep in mind that not all emotional upsets are this easily solved. If your emotional distress is beginning to impact your daily life, consider meeting with a mental health professional in order to assess your condition and make sure that you are getting appropriate treatment that will make you feel better sooner than you could on your own.

Solution: Learn to handle your emotions using non-food related tactics. Include plenty of self-care to help prevent emotional upheaval in the first place.

2. Hydration

The body relies on water to keep joints and organs lubricated and working well, and to add volume for blood to flow throughout our body. Our brain literally cannot function without water. When hydration is not in balance, the body can confuse it with hunger. Dehydration as well as over-hydration triggers hunger due to a lack of available nutrients. When you are dehydrated, certain nutrients do not move as freely throughout the body, and when you are over-hydrated, important nutrients such as sodium, potassium and magnesium are flushed out of the body too quickly.

Generally speaking, people are more likely to be dehydrated than over-hydrated. Many people drink soda instead of water, which does not work as effectively as water to hydrate the body. Soda contains caffeine, which works as a dehydrator, additional sodium, which further dehydrates the body, and sugars, which trigger cravings.

Instead of drinking soda, coffee or even highly caffeinated teas, consider switching to water. Think of this switch like you would a change in your wardrobe from thrifty finds to high-end designer pieces. That's right—wear your water like you do your Prada.

Here's a suggestion to designers out there: why not create beautiful, designer water bottles? Or charms. Fitbit shouldn't be the only healthy accessory adorned by Tory Burch's exquisite designs. Make water fashionable to drink.

Pure water is best, but delicious options are available if you prefer to have some flavor in your drinks. Infuse your water with fruit and herbs. Cut up a lemon or a cucumber and add it to a pitcher of water with some sprigs of mint or slices of ginger to drink all day. Experiment with different options. Come up with your own signature "cocktail."

The transition from drinking sugary, caffeinated beverages to drinking plain water can be tough for some people, but there are ways to achieve it. If you find it difficult, exchange one of your daily sugary drinks for water or flavored water. The next week, exchange another sugary drink for water. By making this transition slowly you will avoid the caffeine crash that can come from dropping caffeine quickly. Eventually, you will find yourself drinking water all day and feeling better than you did when you were drinking sugary, caffeinated beverages.

The formula for appropriate water consumption is to drink half your body weight (pounds) in ounces of water. If you find that you aren't drinking enough water, add an extra glass each week until you are used to drinking the right amount for you. An easy way to get more water is to drink a glass first thing in the morning when you wake up. Add lemon to it to help jumpstart your digestion for the day.

If you find that you need to drink more fluids, try to space the water out over the course of the day. A good boss will set the right pace for any project. Set a recurring alarm on your phone or watch to go off each hour, reminding you to drink a glass of water. Doing so will ensure that you get enough. It will also prevent severe health issues that can arise from drinking too much water at once. Remember to stop drinking at least an hour before bed—two hours would be better—in order to prevent waking up to pee all night.

Some people tend to over-hydrate, which is not good for your body and in extreme cases can lead to serious medical issues. If you are unsure about whether or not you are drinking too much water, track how many ounces of water you drink per day. If you are drinking more than half your body weight in ounces, then you may need to decrease your water intake, depending on your activity levels and environment. Hot yoga, running on the beach, sprinting to a business meeting across 40 city blocks, climbing Mount Everest, or picnicking on Mars may require greater water intake.

Another easy check for hydration is the color of your urine. Dark yellow urine indicates dehydration. Aim for pale yellow or clear (but be aware that clear urine can also indicate over-hydration). Keep in mind that supplements can change the color of your urine as well.

Solution: Take your weight in pounds and cut that number in half. Drink about that much water in ounces per day.

3. Genetics

Our bodies carry the genetic makeup of our parents, grandparents, great grandparents and beyond. Cultural histories, regional influences and individual DNA all contribute to our body's response to food. Over time, imbalances can occur when our bodies react to our personal histories. These imbalances, such as carbohydrate overload or excessive meat consumption, contribute to cravings.

A good boss always does a background check. Not only does the culture you were raised in impact your cravings and the kinds of food you want to eat for comfort, but there are also genetic components that impact how those foods affect your body. Some families are prone to gluten sensitivities, so consuming gluten-heavy meals can cause bloating, gas and discomfort. Certain cultures are also more likely to be lactose intolerant, limiting their consumption of dairy products.

Where you live can have an impact on your cravings, as well. If you live in a place where fatty and carbohydrate-heavy foods are commonplace, it can be hard to resist these foods on a regular basis. Similarly, if your family or peer group has habits that include eating foods that are not in your meal plan, avoiding them will be a challenge. (Avoiding the *foods*, not the family. Ha!)

The best way to steer clear of these genetic and cultural traps is to hold tight to your meal plan and find reasonable substitutes that enable you to participate in the cultural and social events of your family and friends without feeling deprived.

For example, if your background involves eating meat-heavy meals like barbecue, you can make it work by choosing lean meats in reasonable proportions over some of the heavy, fattier dishes that are common at these gatherings.

On the other hand, if your background involves eating a lot of carbohydrates like pasta, you can substitute the pasta for less carbohydrate-heavy options like spaghetti squash or noodles made from beans. You can also substitute buttery, fat-laden sauces for less fattening sauces like arugula pesto or vegetable primavera. Something as simple as a combination of fresh thyme, rosemary, garlic and olive oil can be a perfect accompaniment to the dish.

The important thing to remember when making food choices is that you are not constrained by the foods of your youth or your family. You can make healthier choices even while still having some familiar foods. It might take a little bit of effort to find reasonable substitutes for these foods, but once you do, you can live the rest of your life enjoying your favorite foods in a way that is healthy and balanced.

I lived in Russia the first 20 years of my life. Over the last 16 years, which I've spent in the United States, I have caught myself many times craving foods that I grew up with. I always find a local Russian grocery store in every city I lived in. Russian cuisine is very rich in dairy and fermented foods, which happen to be good sources of protein and probiotics, or beneficial bacteria. Of course, there are some junk foods available, too. Every once in a while I allow myself to connect with my roots and indulge.

Solution: Accept that genetics are a factor when it comes to your cravings, and use what you know from your family history and cultural background to make the best decisions that you can for yourself. Get creative with new renditions of old recipes.

4. Changes in seasons

We've all heard the term *winter fat*. Winter fat accumulates when you eat certain foods in order to compensate for things like seasonal depression, inactivity or to alleviate boredom from being cooped up inside due to frigid temperatures.

Just like creatures in the animal kingdom that store up fatty foods to add a warm layer of fat to last throughout the long winter season, we also tend to be more attracted to heartier choices, especially if we live in cold climates.

The food choices we go for during winter are soups, stews, pies and starchy vegetables—it all goes in perfect harmony with the holiday season. For those of us living in the United States, Halloween becomes the biggest day of sugar overdose, followed by a total stuffing—literally—during Thanksgiving dinner. Then comes December with holiday party after party.

How can we avoid all the delicious food served during the holidays?

One popular trick is to eat a healthy meal before you go to the party so that you are not hungry when you arrive. I recommend eating a small meal so that you can still participate—just be sure to choose the healthier foods that are offered.

Another option is to plan ahead and think about what will be served. You are likely to see the same dishes year in and year out. Many families serve the same dishes every year for Thanksgiving. If you know you are about to have a faceoff with sweet potato pie, plan to pass that dish when it comes around or simply take a small taste if passing it up might offend your host.

Yet another option, and one of my personal favorites, is to offer to bring a dish to the party. This way, you know for sure that there will be at least one dish at the party that suits your diet and that you will enjoy.

Above all, beware of the drinks at these parties. From eggnog and mulled wine to endless bowls of mystery punch, holiday beverages are a bottomless pit of calories and sugar that is only going to increase your cravings. I don't want you to feel deprived because you can't enjoy your favorite holiday beverage, but I do want you to be a boss about it. Have a single glass of your favorite holiday drink and sip it slowly. Then, switch to water to help keep you hydrated and prevent the consumption of unwanted sugar and calories. Or don't drink alcohol at all – as a pleasant bonus, you can drive home safely at the end of the night.

As though holiday parties weren't enough, the bigger issue involves the meals you eat alone in the winter. You know what I mean—that comfort food that only manages to make you *less comfortable* in your new jeans. There is a hard limit to how many heavy stews, creamy sauces, and chicken pot pies you can consume before you have to pull out your fat jeans. Be sure to recognize that limit before it's too late.

A good boss gets creative with solutions. You can find lighter versions of almost any dish available online. Don't feel daunted by the idea of having to figure out how to make your favorite meals healthy—rest assured that someone has beaten you to it. The Internet is a marvelous thing. Get searching, boss!

It's not likely that you will completely eliminate heavy meals from your winter menu. I wouldn't ask you to. But I will ask you to limit how many of these meals you consume. Plan to have one or two every week, and continue to eat as you did during summer for the rest of your meals. It's the best of both worlds.

Solution: *Change your mindset to "winter skinny." Get creative with holiday parties. Seek out healthy options, bring your own dish, and keep your indulgences to a minimum.*

5. Stress

Stress can cause an increase or decrease in the production of digestive enzymes and stomach acids. It can also tempt you to soothe yourself by eating comfort foods. Stress wreaks havoc on your digestion and elimination processes and adds unhealthy, unwanted calories.

The pervasive nature of stress is one of the greatest problems in society today. Ask anyone how they feel and the answer is almost always some variation of, "I'm really stressed. I'm really busy." Not only do we tend to over-schedule ourselves, but in many families, each family member has a complicated and varying schedule that must be coordinated and worked around.

Add to that the seemingly inevitable pressures of work and conflicts in personalities with co-workers and family members, and it's no wonder that we all seem to be far more stressed than we used to be.

The way to solve this problem without adding to the stress or to your waistline is to follow a simple evaluation system. First, sit down and take a long look at your life. What is causing the most stress? Which areas are problematic? Once you identify stressors, you can begin to look for the trigger moments.

For example, you may feel stressed because you can never seem to stay on top of your housework. You come home from a hard day of work followed by shuttling your children to and from soccer; then comes homework and—oh yeah, *dinner*—and you still have a basket full of laundry to contend with. Your stress level peaks at the sight of that basket.

A good boss strategizes. Evaluate your housework plan, and make small changes that make your situation easier. Perhaps you delegate by encouraging your family members to take over some household chores. Or maybe you implement a no-clutter rule so the mess doesn't accumulate as the week goes on. Implement a new strategy and get your team (family, that is) on board.

Solution: *Evaluate your stress areas, learn your triggers, and make one small change per week.*

6. Inadequate intake of nutrients

If you are not providing your body with the nutrients it requires to perform basic functions, cravings become a way for the body to communicate its needs. A diet high in sugar, bad fats and processed foods creates imbalances that rob the body of energy and essential nutrients.

Let's look at this example: You buy a poor quality briefcase made by a machine at a factory in some faraway land only to have something break off every week. Would you buy another one to save money and time in the short-term or would you invest in a high-quality bag that prevents your important documents from falling out and landing in a puddle when the bag breaks again?

This is exactly what it's like to choose foods with high nutritional value—they will serve the body for much longer, unlike foods made by machines in faraway lands.

The solution is simple to implement but often hard to maintain over time. Begin by logging all the foods you eat and drinks you consume in an app or a dedicated journal that you carry with you all the time. Don't make any dietary changes at first. Just make sure to log every single bite you take.

After a couple of weeks of logging all your meals and all your drinks, the imbalances will become clear to you. While you may not eat all the nutrients you should every day, over a period of a couple of weeks a quality picture or a pattern will emerge, and you can take a wider view of your eating habits. At that point, it may be clear that you aren't eating enough vegetables or getting enough protein. Or maybe you're eating more sugar than you thought.

One of the advantages of using one of the many free food-tracking apps available for your phone is that most of them track not only calories but also nutrients like sugar, sodium, protein, etc. Some will even track your activity levels—or inactivity, as the case may be. Using an app to track your diet and habits will make it easier to understand what changes you need to make.

Remember: You can't act upon what you can't measure.

A good boss is always aware of the numbers. Tracking your food intake and activity is like balancing your checkbook. Is the money coming in equal to the money going out? Are you eating foods with high nutritional value? Does your body metabolize effectively? Are you getting enough exercise?

Most of us tend to eat the same handful of meals over and over. Tracking your meals can give you some insight into whether or not those meals need to be modified or replaced to give you a healthier balance of nutrients.

By gradually, intentionally, steadily, progressively and consistently making better dietary choices you will get the benefit of proper nutritional balance. The amount of time it takes to see the benefits vary from person to person and depends upon whether you have an existing nutritional deficiency and if so, how severe it is.

> *"Nutrients work together as does an orchestra. Like instruments playing in harmony, all the nutrients must be available in their optimum amounts." —Adapted from Dr. Roger Williams*

Inadequate intake of nutrients will eventually lead to nutrient deficiencies, especially when it comes to vitamins and minerals. Now, before you cringe at the thought of having to think about the periodic table, relax. We are not going to go all the way back to your chemistry class. Besides, I don't know about you, but those weren't good hair days for me. Let's keep the past right where it belongs: in the past.

Lack of specific vitamins and minerals is potentially one of the most overlooked causes of cravings. In fact, sometimes the simplest solutions involve the implementation of megavitamin therapies.

For example, many women crave chocolate right before their period due to a magnesium deficiency, according to Carolyn Dean, MD, ND, author of *Magnesium Miracle*.[9] Chocolate is a great source of magnesium. However, according to the Institute for Functional Medicine's book *Clinical Nutrition*, the top five sources of magnesium are kelp, wheat bran, wheat germ, almonds and cashews.

In the book *Putting it All Together: The New Orthomolecular Nutrition*, authors Abram Hoffer, MD, PhD and Morton Walker, DPM shed a lot of light on these types of therapies. "The basic or fundamental rule of orthomolecular . . . care today is to depend on optimum doses of nutrients most likely to help the patient recover."

A lack of certain nutrients will not only cause general functional abnormalities, but may cause very specific cravings. See the table below to get an idea about whether nutrient deficiencies may be at the root of your cravings. If you suspect so, follow up with your doctor to get blood work to confirm.

Solution: *Track all your food and drinks in a journal or app to find imbalances that you can correct.*

IF YOU ARE CRAVING THIS	WHAT YOUR BODY IS LACKING	TRY THIS INSTEAD
Breads, Pasta, Refined Carbs	Nitrogen	Lean animal protein, fish, legumes.
Chocolate, Sour Food	Magnesium	Kelp, wheat bran, raw nuts, buckwheat. Try soaking in Epsom salt bath.
Carbonated Drinks Fatty Food	Calcium	Kelp, Swiss/cheddar cheese, sardines, sesame seeds, collard/turnip greens, almonds, parsley.
Cold Drinks	Manganese	Raw nuts, barley, buckwheat, fresh spinach.
Salty Food	Chloride	Kelp, fish, unrefined sea salt, olives, sauerkraut, fresh goat milk.
Sweets	Chromium	Meats, whole grains, oysters.
	Vanadium	Buckwheat, parsley, safflower oil, eggs.
Coffee/Tea	Iron	Kelp, Brewer's yeast, pumpkin/sunflower seeds, beef liver, parsley.
	Sulphur	Eggs, meats, legumes.
Ice	Iron	Kelp, Brewer's yeast, pumpkin/sunflower seeds, beef liver, parsley.
*No Appetite	Vitamins B1	Brewer's yeast, sunflower seeds, pine nuts, peanuts, pecans.
	Vitamins B2	Brewer's yeast, liver, almonds.
*Always Hungry	Tryptophan	Nuts and seeds, seaweed, spinach, shellfish, soy, game, chicken, turkey, fish, oats, beans, lentils, and eggs.
	Tyrosine	Cheese, soybeans, beef, lamb, pork, fish, chicken, nuts, seeds, eggs, beans.

★Ask your doctor to do blood work to confirm deficiencies.

7. Hormonal imbalances

For women, hormonal imbalances occur during monthly cycles, pregnancy and menopause, but they can also occur at other times. For men, life changes and advancing age can contribute to low testosterone levels. Hormone imbalances such as these can add to cravings.

A woman's body changes throughout each monthly cycle, sometimes dramatically, and these changes often bring cravings. During certain times of the month, you might feel bloated and heavy, not wanting to eat much, while during other parts of the month you might find yourself unusually hungry or craving specific foods, often salty or sugary treats.

Creating hormonal harmony requires a delicate balance between respecting the needs of the body and being cautious about overindulgence. Generally speaking, if you are aware of these phases in your life, you should be able to plan for them and arrange your life accordingly. That doesn't mean you can never have something sweet or chocolaty during your cycle; rather, it means that you should know that your craving is caused by hormones and not a biological imperative. This knowledge can help you to resist the craving and stick to your eating plan. However, if you do allow yourself a certain amount of sugar per week or per month, you can allocate those sweets for these times to ensure that you get the comfort you need without throwing your eating plan off balance.

Men often find that as they get older, their tastes and appetites change. But many men continue to eat as they did during the teenage years, even when their metabolism and lifestyle no longer support that level of consumption. When men understand that their food intake must decrease naturally over time, they will be better able to avoid the weight gain that often settles in during middle age. Making systematic and gradual changes is the best approach for men.

Solution: *Recognize your hormone cycles and imbalances so that you can anticipate them and plan ahead. Be knowledgeable and proactive.*

8. Sensory stimulation

Your senses are constantly in evaluation mode of your surroundings, taking in sights, sounds, smells, tastes and textures so that the body can understand how to behave in its environment. What your senses take in can affect your food cravings. In fact, researchers of the Max Planck Society have shown that even images of food stimulate appetite.[10] Think about how the food industry spends billions of dollars on marketing and creating commercials that literally make you drool. Before you know it, you're on your ninth cookie or worse—on your way to the nearest fast food restaurant while under the spell. Cravings are known to interfere with cognitive functioning, partly because they use the same parts of the brain. That explains the sensory-induced trance.

Visual stimulation makes total sense when you think of being seduced by piles of cashmere, boots and sweaters in the fall, or bathing suits and little dresses in the spring.

Anyone who has ever said, "Oh, I'm not hungry. You go ahead and eat," to their partner only to wander into the kitchen wondering what smells so good and asking if there's enough to share has experienced this phenomenon firsthand. Or what about pizza at the office on Friday afternoon? There you are sitting at your desk, minding your own business when the pizza delivery fairy walks past, trailing an undeniable scent of cheesy perfection. Suddenly, you are "starving" and must remedy your famine with four slices. Forget the healthy lunch you packed in your cooler. It's pizza time. Not to mention the two birthday cakes this week. Or maybe your downfall is popcorn at the movies. Sure, you'll upgrade to a super-duper size for a dollar—what a deal! Or what about, "Look, it's the UPS guy! Let's celebrate his delivery of my long-awaited shoes I had no business blowing my salary on." Yeah, we've been there. The distractions are endless.

Have you ever noticed that during dinnertime, advertisers run ad after ad for restaurants? They know that if you see their burgers, you are more likely to grab the keys and head on over. They are appealing to your senses because it works.

A good boss takes time to get to know her market. In this case, knowledge is power. Once you know for a fact that you are being manipulated by your brain, you can start to change the hold it has over you. When you smell pizza and get hungry, stop. Say to yourself, "I do not need to eat that pizza. I have already eaten a balanced and healthy meal, and I know that my brain is tricking me into hunger."

I have a great tip. Find a natural essential oil that you like and tuck it into your pocket. When you feel a sensory urge come on, take a whiff of the oil to create a diversion. I like peppermint or rosemary best—they are very invigorating. At home, keep pots of fresh herbs in your kitchen. Rub the fresh leaves in your hands and at the base of your nose when you feel a craving come on.

Getting the buy-in and participation of your family members is also key. If you can't sit in the house while your family eats pizza or freshly baked cinnamon rolls without feeling miserable, convince your family to eat pizza and pastries elsewhere—or not at all. They deserve healthy, balanced nutritional meals too. And there are many healthy pizza recipes out there! For non-compliant family members buy a locked cabinet to keep their junk food locked away. That way you won't continue to lose the staring contest with cheese puffs.

Keeping the junk food outside of arm's reach will force you to make better choices. Add five healthy options to your fridge or pantry, and always make them your first choice.

You could also simply leave the room and go for a five-minute walk. Take the garbage out or walk the dog. Call a friend. Take a bath. Look at your vision board. Eat an apple. Plant a tree. Make silly faces at yourself in the mirror. Play tic-tac-toe. Get a manicure. Rearrange furniture. Memorize a short poem. You get the picture.

Solution: *Get rid of or lock up all your "weakness" foods. Create distraction techniques to take your mind off the sensory overload. Come up with a reward system for sticking to your goals.*

9. Carryover flavors

Your tongue is covered with taste buds that provide continuing nerve stimulation. If there are leftover food particles on the tongue, the desire to keep that taste in the mouth will cause continued cravings.

This seems like an insurmountable obstacle in the face of it. You are not always in a place where you can brush your teeth. How are you supposed to solve this problem?

The first way, and the easiest, is to drink water after you eat, swishing the water around in your mouth to get out as many of the leftover food particles as possible. You can do this anywhere with no problem at all. The only real downside is that it isn't a foolproof method. There will likely still be some food particles left when you swish with water.

A good boss has to think outside the box. The second option requires a strange but useful tool and a little bit more time and commitment but will get rid of most or all of the leftover food particles. It involves the almighty tongue scraper. Yes, I am asking you to scrape your tongue after every meal. It may sound silly, but it will help you get rid of virtually all the leftover food particles, eliminating them as a source of your cravings. Go purchase a tongue scraper and carry it with you. Trust me on this one. You may get funny glances in the bathroom, but it's absolutely worth it.

Solution: A tongue scraper is the most helpful tool to remove food particles from your tongue that trigger food cravings.

10. Opposites attract

When you excessively consume a certain type of food, or engage in long strenuous activity, the body will want to balance itself out by producing a desire for the opposite. For example, if you go for a long run on the beach in the heat, your body will want to cool itself and demand cooling foods and beverages like water or fruit. If you eat too much sweet food, your body will "ask" for salty, bitter or sour flavors. You have blond straight hair, you want dark and curly. Ummm this is a whole other topic.

This makes handling cravings fairly simple. If you find that you are craving sweet foods, you can look back at your food journal or your food app (you are keeping a food journal, right?) to see if you have been eating an unusually high amount of bitter, sour or salty foods. If you have, your craving is explained.

The way to eliminate cravings is by understanding them. You can't just stop cravings without first trying to understand their messages. That's what I'm trying to have you wrap your head around. Your food journal or app is the solution. When you find yourself craving a certain type of food on a regular basis, keep a closer eye on your food habits.

By checking your food journal each night, you can see these imbalances when they start. If you look at the day and see that you have eaten more sugar than you should have, the next day you can avoid it.

A good boss looks for patterns. By paying attention to your patterns, you will get into a more balanced eating system over time so that imbalances like these almost never happen.

Solution: Take note of the patterns in your cravings for certain foods so that you can even out your eating habits to avoid craving opposite flavors.

11. Lack of sleep

Matthew Walker, PhD, a UC Berkeley researcher and professor of psychology and neuroscience stated, "High-calorie foods also became significantly more desirable when participants were sleep-deprived. This combination of altered brain activity and decision-making may help explain why people who sleep less also tend to be overweight or obese."[11,12]

A sleepless night will not only impair your decision-making processes, make you more grouchy and deteriorate your overall health, but it will also make you more likely to reach for doughnuts or candy rather than for whole grains or leafy green vegetables. Studies find that sleep deprivation can make us crave junk food more than healthy choices.

You have almost certainly had the experience of staying up too late and then having to get up early the next morning. Remember your college days? You wake up feeling terrible exhaustion. On a normal day you might have a healthy and balanced breakfast—perhaps some oatmeal and fruit sprinkled with nuts—but this day you are suddenly craving a doughnut or pastries. Or a bloody Mary. Or cold, leftover pizza. Or waffles piled high with bacon and maple syrup. Or you might find yourself pulling through the drive-through about to order a greasy breakfast.

Sleep problems have become more pervasive as we try to cram more and more activities and work into a finite amount of time. Between work, children's homework and activities, housework, personal projects and fitness, there is hardly any time to spend on ourselves. Everyone and everything takes priority. Too many people sacrifice the time they could be sleeping in order to complete projects or get some time for themselves or with their partner.

In addition, the stress we discussed earlier can impede your ability to fall asleep because you stay up thinking about the problems in your life. And once you get to sleep, you'll probably sleep poorly. That constant chatter in your brain needs to rest. Problems don't get resolved while lying in bed worrying.

A good boss creates routines. As hard as it may be, disciplined and focused sleep habits are vital. Good sleep practice is simple, but it requires follow-through. Be sure to use your bed only for sleeping and "under the sheets" activities; turn off anything with a screen at least two hours before bed (I'm looking at your social media); engage in calm and relaxing activities before you go to sleep; eliminate any light sources from entering your bedroom; and don't eat within a couple hours of bedtime.

Beyond that, it is important to go to sleep and get up at the same time each day. Although most of us use weekends to catch up on sleep, this does more harm than good for us in the long term. If you find that you can't get to sleep at a regular time because of your commitments, try to eliminate or outsource them in order to get the sleep you need.

Self-care is not self*fish*. When you are in an airplane, they tell you to put on your own oxygen mask first if there's an emergency. Your self-care is like that oxygen mask. We have to keep ourselves in functional shape or we are of minimal use to our family members and coworkers.

Solution: *Establish good sleep routines to avoid the next-morning craving trap.*

12. Habit

If you are reading this, you have probably found yourself seeking the affection of chocolate kisses, staring at the bottom of a bag of pretzels, or grabbing a daily doughnut on autopilot. "The car literally turned into the drive-through!" Habits are learned behaviors, which mean that there are strategies to break them if you become truly aware and pay attention. Your every experience with food should be conscious, not automatic.

Habits are powerful. For some reason good habits are less sticky, but only if we haven't familiarized ourselves with the full benefits package. When was the last time you heard someone say, "I'm in the habit of doing squats while blow-drying my hair?" There are many different ways to make a habit work *for* you instead of *against* you. In fact, because studies have shown that we have a finite store of willpower, the best way to develop a powerful life and to meet your goals is to develop positive habits.

Much like the automatic fast food visit, you can also automatically reprogram your body to eat nothing but good foods. Start your day with a green smoothie, or prepare something nutritious the night before.

The most effective people in our society are those who have habits that automate their proactive and positive life choices.

For example, although forming the habit of exercise is difficult, once in place it's fairly easy to maintain. You don't have to make the decision to get up and run before work because you *always* get up and run before work. It's just what you do. Similarly, if you make the habit to shut off your electronic devices, have a warm bath or shower, and go to bed at the same time each night, it's easy for you to continue to do so because you no longer have to think about it.

The hard part is forming the habit in the first place. Instead of trying to break existing bad habits, make an effort to replace bad habits with positive ones that improve the quality of your life. Let's face it: your daily coffee and pastry habit is really just expensive and detrimental to your health. Why not replace it with a positive habit of waking up and making a delicious, nutrient-filled smoothie? In order to cement this habit, consider taking a different path to work every day so you are no longer driving past your usual coffee shop.

By automating your positive habits, like fitness, and by making a habit to eat at home and pack your lunch, you are making conscious decisions about what is going into your body. Instead of allowing previous bad habits to dictate your actions, you can be a boss and take control of your choices. Eventually, with time and practice, you can swing the power of habit in a positive direction and have a new pattern of healthy, balanced eating without the struggle of deciding what foods to eat at every meal.

Solution: *Begin to replace your bad habits with positive ones. Read "The Power of Habit" by Charles Dohigg to understand why habits exist and how they can be changed. Pick up a new hobby to replace a bad habit.*

13. Wandering mind

Could it be that your cravings are the result of simple boredom? An idle mind will look for anything to keep itself engaged. The brain can't function without food, so it will constantly ask for refills, especially when unoccupied. While it may not be the worst thing to allow your mind to wander at times, sort through thoughts, contemplate events and allow space for creativity, you don't want junk food to become the daily accessory. Stick to shoes and handbags.

Unconscious eating is a major problem for many people. How many times have you sat in front of the television with a bag of chips, maybe watching a sports match? By the end of the game the bag is empty. You didn't mean to eat all the chips, and you certainly should not have eaten an entire bag, but you were so busy watching the game that you didn't realize that you were eating enough chips to feed the entire sports team. Similarly, have you ever eaten an entire tub of theater popcorn by the end of the movie—an entire day's worth of calories? Did you intend to eat all that popcorn? Not likely.

Or maybe you find yourself with some free time. You have no projects to complete and nothing to do. You wander around your house, restless. Should you read a book? Watch a movie? Do a puzzle? The next thing you know, you're in the kitchen, rummaging through the refrigerator or pantry.

A good boss pays attention to the task at hand. If you have a habit of mindless snacking in front of the television, portion out your snacks before you sit down. Measure out as many as you intend to eat or, even better, get some vegetables instead and eat the exact amount you portioned out before you get to the couch.

If you tend to mindlessly snack when you are bored, make a list of things you can do when you have some available minutes or hours, enjoyable things like walking the dog, painting, gardening, sewing, dancing, tutoring, learning to play a violin, watching a show about animals, creating a vision board, reading a book, dancing naked around the house, balancing your checkbook, making a list of local charities, writing out thank you cards, organizing your pantry or volunteering your time to someone who could really use it. Then, when you have some free time you won't feel like you are at loose ends. Instead, you can go directly to the list of activities you made and feel like you are making the most of your time.

Solution: Set aside certain times a day for meditation or mindless wandering. You could listen to a podcast, read a book, or talk to a friend. During other times, be deliberate about your actions.

14. Changes in brain chemistry

Mark Gold, MD, a researcher at the University of Florida, presented summaries of brain imaging research at several leading universities showing that "palatable food," or very tasty food, creates the same types of changes in the dopamine receptors of the human brain as alcohol and other widely recognized addictive substances. Multiple researches have shown that sugar and other sweets activate the same reward and addiction centers of the brain as cocaine as I mentioned earlier. There is also research showing that out-of-control consumption of food may be due to the body's need to reduce pain, based on serotonin mechanisms in the brain.

If you have been eating a lot of sweet foods, you will likely find that if you suddenly stop eating sugar, you have intense sugar cravings. This is not a surprise, as evidenced by the research cited above. Sugar works on the brain like an addictive substance. It triggers withdrawal symptoms that cause cravings.

Parts of the brain will receive a delayed message that you have consumed food, which is especially dangerous for people with food addictions who will continue to fuel the pleasure centers of their brain with foods. This can create a real catastrophe:

Your brain sees the food, you have an uncontrollable desire to consume it, and you eat too much because the body doesn't recognize that it's had enough.

It isn't just as simple as stepping away from the cookies, though. It requires diligence. Check the labels on your favorite foods. Many of them have some form of sugar in them. Spaghetti sauce, salad dressing and even frozen dinners have added sugars. You are likely getting more sugar in your system than you realize.

The high amounts of fat in fast food and other processed food is similarly addictive. Many of these foods also have added sugar, making it a nasty double-edged sword. Breaking the cycle of addiction to fatty and sugary foods might seem insurmountable, but it isn't. However, it's important to understand that it will feel like breaking an addiction to cigarettes or alcohol—it's a challenge. Go slowly and give yourself some leeway.

Although some people find that going cold turkey on these foods is the easiest way to break the cycle of addiction, in many other cases, a gradual reduction of the amount of added fats and sugars that you consume while introducing new, more nutritional alternatives, will make it easier to break your addiction.

A good boss knows when it's time to change course and when to call for help if needed. If you find that you can't do it by yourself, consider getting support from an organization that is equipped to help you, like Overeaters Anonymous.

Solution: *Recognizing that simple cravings can create serious food addictions requires a strong commitment and may require intervention from organizations like Overeaters Anonymous. Ultimately, temporary food abstinence relieves physical craving over time.*

15. Social disconnect

We are meant to be social creatures. Positive, meaningful interactions enrich our lives with joy and purpose. Feelings of loneliness often lead to mind traps. Self-criticism, thoughts like, "I'm not loved," or "I'm not good enough," have a way of overtaking our minds. This in turn leads to the desire to turn to food for comfort.

This is the truest form of "eating your feelings." You feel empty inside so you try to fill the void with food. This never works. Not only are you still lonely and disconnected, but you also end up feeling guilty and disappointed in yourself. The thoughts in your head go from, "What does it matter if I eat or not?" to "I have no self-control or discipline," making the overall situation much worse than if you had not eaten at all.

In order to solve the problem, you must address it at the source. The food isn't the problem, loneliness is. The social connections you have in your life determine, in part, your ability to handle life's stresses. The more social connections you have, the more likely you are to cope with life's upsets.

The reverse, of course, is also true. The less social connections you have, the harder it is for you to handle life's stresses and the more likely you are to engage in eating to fill the void in your heart.

A good boss knows the value of community. Muster up a surge of courage and fortitude and put yourself out there to forge new connections. You will reap massive rewards over time. While making new friends may seem like something you did only in your youth, there are several ways to make friends and start to reverse the loneliness in your life.

Consider joining a club. Many cities have groups and organizations for many different interests listed online that meet at regular intervals. If you are interested in board games or video games, there are gaming groups available in many cities. If you prefer outdoor activities, there are hiking groups and cycling groups, as well as running groups. You name it—a group for it probably exists near you. If not, start one!

Another source of social interaction is local religious organizations. Although many people are raised in a faith as a child, far fewer adults are involved in their local religious group. Consider trying out a church, synagogue, mosque or whatever place of religious expression applies to you. These organizations not only have weekly services that get you out of the house and meeting new people, but they also have events outside of regular services, from trivia nights and music events to outings that visit local tourist attractions or restaurants.

Finally, consider taking a course through your local community college or recreation department. Many recreation departments offer a wide range of classes from sports to crafting.

You can pursue an interest and meet other people who are interested in the same activities as you.

No matter what you choose, getting out there and finding a group of people with whom you can socialize will improve your life in many different areas—not only your food consumption, but also your emotional life.

Solution: *Sometimes all it takes is taking one step outside your comfort zone and towards healthy relationships. Surrounding yourself with loving, supportive people will fill in the gap caused by loneliness.*

Are you feeding your body or nourishing it?

STEP 3. PINPOINT THE TRIGGER

Picture this scenario: You have a really stressful day at work. At the end of the day all you want is something sweet to activate the "feel good" center of your brain. Triggers play a very important role, and can sometimes be the primary differentiating factor between adding an extra 1,000 calories to your daily budget. Let's explore some triggers of food cravings:

Triggers can be *external* (activities, situations, events and things you encounter in the environment).

Or *internal* (feelings, emotions and thoughts).

One of the most interesting things I learned from the Institute for Functional Medicine is that there's always a trigger behind every change in behavior. ***Whether you consciously realize it or not, single or multiple triggers have the power of sending you into self-destructing behaviors.*** And not just with your food choices.

True behavior modification techniques are easier to incorporate than you think once the problems are identified.

Think of the causes discussed earlier in this book **as processes** that have made you susceptible to cravings over time. **Triggers are specific events** that make you eat certain foods at a particular point in time. The central idea here is that the combination of causes and a trigger creates the crisis of indulgence.

Take the cause of visual stimulation for example. We are always surrounded by it—commercials on TV, print ads, food packaging, enticing pies and pastries behind bakery displays. Yet we do not rip open the packages and devour snacks while walking through the aisles of the grocery store. But at one particular moment in time our defenses go down, and we are triggered by a certain commercial or the bourbon chicken offered at a food court. Our brains go on high alert and send signals telling us to eat NOW.

Trigger ID questionnaire.

To help you identify your triggers, answer the following questions:

☐ Do you feel a craving always come on in certain environments, certain times of day or around certain people? _____

_____

☐ What feelings trigger your cravings? _____

_____

☐ How can you be more mindful of these triggers so that you don't fall prey to your cravings? _____

_____

Now that you have identified your triggers, think about which are avoidable and which are not.

How can you successfully manage your triggers?

☐ Try distraction.
☐ Ride it out.
☐ Get support.
☐ Your own solution:

_____

_____

_____

_____

STEP 4. PROMOTE YOUR IMAGINATION

This is the fun part. Now you get to take your imagination where it wants to go. Visualizing your potential outcome will rewire your initial brain response.

Here is a fun little exercise. Pretend that in front of you stands your Hollywood crush, asking you to go for a walk on the beach. Or envision that you just got a call to be in a Victoria's Secret fashion show. Maybe you're giving a speech to young kids about how to eat so they have more energy. Maybe you envision yourself having enough stamina to explore Machu Picchu. Or maybe you want to look extra hot on a date with that special someone you've been with for 20 years. Wherever your imagination takes you, make it really fun and outrageous.

When you visualize your ideal (or in this case fantasy) scenario, how does that change your response to a triggered craving? What would you do at that moment? Would you fall face forward and devour the birthday cake or would you have a polite bite and later do 15 jumping jacks while telling yourself, "I love you?"

Let your fantasy come out to play here. Imagine the wildest scenario—the one that will push you toward realizing your goals.

An innovative boss always knows where to turn for creative ways to solve problems—how will you engage your intellect?

ARRANGE YOUR ENVIRONMENT FOR SUCCESS

Which office would you prefer: the one in the big corner, tidy, with lots of light and room to breathe, or a desk that you can barely see with piles of papers of every color and scattered with gum and candy wrappers stuck to quarterly reports?

Arranging your environment for success will help you more intentionally and purposefully make decisions and take actions.

1. If you know that it's extremely difficult for you to give into temptations of chocolate covered bacon flavored potato chips, get rid of them.
2. Keep healthy snacks on hand at any given moment. Download my list of 25 intentionally healthy snacks here: http://healthy-intent.com/newsletter/

3. Announce to everyone that you have been promoted. You are now the boss of your cravings. You'd be surprised how supporting people around you will be. And many will want to join you.

4. Be ready to engage in non-food related rewards.

STEP 5 – "FIRE YOUR CRAVINGS" ACTION WORKSHEETS

These worksheets are available for download at <u>www.cravingsboss.com/</u> <u>resources</u>

1. Change your reward system.

Most of us can probably admit to using food as a reward. From the birthday cake you received each year beginning at age one and the ice cream treats and lollipops you enjoyed after earning high marks on your report card or visiting the dentist to the sweet treat you allow yourself after a workout, this system has been a part of your life since you can remember.

It's now on you to break the patterns.

The idea is to transition to non-food related rewards, thus rewiring your brain to desire an activity rather than empty calories.

Think of activities that bring you joy. Go back to your childhood if you have to. Write them down. Make sure to come up with a couple completely random, unexpected and fun rewards and experiences.

_____

_____

Make a list of how you WANT to feel after eating:

_____

_____

The point here is to refocus your thoughts away from deprivation and towards healthy rewards.

Remember the reward chart you had as a kid? Maybe it's time to bring it back, but for your behavior.

2. Cravings ID worksheet

		MY CRAVINGS JOURNAL			
Date	Time	What	Where	Thoughts/Feelings	My Response

www.cravingsboss.com/resources
w   www.healthyintent.com   e   info@healthy-intent.com

3. Cravings action ID worksheet

1. Affirmations

Pick several statements that might help you avoid giving into cravings:

- ☐ My health is more important to me than . . .[ice cream, chips, etc.]
- ☐ I will make smart decisions today.
- ☐ Other:

_____

_____

2. Distractions

Pick an activity that will shift the focus off your craving:

- ☐ Listen to music
- ☐ Garden
- ☐ Write in your journal
- ☐ Go for a walk/run
- ☐ Call or text a friend or supporter
- ☐ Do a breathing exercise
- ☐ Other:

_____

_____

5-STEP PLAN REVIEW

Let's review your new plan:

1. Have a two-minute board meeting with yourself. Don't act on the craving immediately. Pause for two minutes.
2. Examine the facts. Figure out the underlying cause. Remember what you've learned.
3. Pinpoint the trigger. What exactly is threatening to take away your power at that particular moment?
4. Promote your imagination. Visualize the outcome.
5. Fire those cravings. Take action that will lead you to your ideal outcome.

Now that you understand why your craving exists and you have the inspiration for making changes that last, put it into action. You're in charge, boss. Choose a food that feeds your health, not your waistline. Or choose an activity that feeds your soul. Make any one of the many choices offered to you in this book.

MY SECRET WEAPONS

The health coach in me wants to tell you about the importance of mindset. You can literally think your way out of your cravings. Shift your focus to another activity. Turn on some fun music, dance, and create any kind of diversion.

I like to pass my time in the following ways: zentangling, crocheting, working on an art project with my daughter, writing poetry, and having a stimulating conversation with my husband or friends.

I have also learned to always keep some kind of a snack on hand. I find it easy to have a little bag of mixed nuts and seeds in my purse at all times. I feel like I'm part squirrel some days, but popping a few nuts into my mouth has saved me on many different occasions.

All you need is a tiny bag with a dozen or so nuts and a few seeds in it. Nuts are rich in protein, vitamin E, and healthy fats.

While some people have certain nut allergies, I find that most people can keep this simple snack on hand. Think of an easy and healthy portable snack you can always have on hand for those "extreme cravings emergencies."

One more trick. I always keep a shaker bottle with me filled with vegan protein powder. Just add water and ice and voilà! Instant protein shake.

CONCLUSION

Every day we are faced with important decisions. Life-changing decisions. Why should the decision of what to eat be secondary?

Cravings may have had power over you in the past, but it's time for you to take charge.

Now you know how to tell the difference between hunger and cravings; understand the effects of sugar and salt; recognize the many causes of cravings; be aware of the triggers; and most important, to take action in many different situations.

You have all the power to turn your cravings around. One day at a time. One small change per week. Consistently. Over time, with practice, you will look back to today and think: "Wow! I have come so far. I have a healthy body, and I make conscious decisions about what I eat."

Read out loud: "I am the boss of my cravings!"

No matter what you do, aim for your end result to positive thinking without guilt. Your body needs quality fuel to function well. Do right by it, and it will serve you as a reliable vessel for many happy years. You've got this! You are stronger than any craving that comes your way. The only thing separating you from winning the battle with cravings for good is your choice.

BE A CRAVINGS BOSS!

ENDNOTES

How do you feel at this point? What are your thoughts? Do you feel more confident? Are you ready to dive into the worksheets and get to know yourself?

More importantly, *what are you going to do about your cravings?*

Remember that understanding the causes of your cravings is only a small part of the big picture. As you read through the fifteen causes of cravings, maybe just one or several things jumped out at you. Going beyond each cause can be an emotional moment. Please know that I am here for you every step of the way.

So many scenarios arise during my coaching sessions with clients. I've helped them face raw emotions and heal through conversation and openness. *My main goals are to create a safe space for open communication, and to come up with a plan to move forward.*

My eight-week long Vital Life program helps people better understand the concepts presented in this book. It is designed to give you the tools to eliminate self-sabotaging behaviors and transform your ways of looking at challenging, energy-draining situations.

One of the main complaints I hear from my clients is, "I am always tired." In today's world, ample amounts of energy are needed to keep up with ever-increasing lifestyle demands. Vital Life educates you about foods and behaviors that drain energy and those that give you energy. High-energy individuals always seem to accomplish more and have better and healthier relationships with themselves and others. That's what Vital Life is all about.

Look out for the discount code on the next page.

CRAVING MORE?

VITAL LIFE – Your 8-week unique path to personal well-being.

Get ready to learn step-by-step how to optimize your cellular energy production through food, exercise and lifestyle adjustments.

Learn more at www.healthy-intent.com/vital-life

Use code HI15OFF to get 15% off on Vital Life program.

Come hang out with Healthy Intent on Social media:

www.facebook.com/hiintent   *https://instagram.com/*   *@*
                                healthy_intent   *hihealthyintent*

I'd like to extend special thanks to everyone supporting me during the process of creating of this book.

Joanne Steinheardt – you have been my inspiration, always challenging me to produce my best work.

Natalie Diasti – thank you for always cheering me on with your sense of humor.

Nat Guy – so grateful for your mentorship.

Heidi Hapanowicz – you are the most talented photographer. Thank you for the amazing pictures.

Jamey Jones – thank you for your countless hours of editing.

My husband Mark – without you planting the idea of publishing a book in my head, this would have been a long blog post.

Did you like this book? I'd love your feedback.

Email me at: info@healthy-intent.com

With Love,

NATALIA LEVEY
Cravings Boss

NOTES

1   http://foodaddictioninstitute.org/scientific-research/physical-craving-and-food-addiction-a-scientific-review/ Accessed 11/05/2015.

2   Cohen DL and Townsend RR, "The salt controversy and hypertension." *J Clin Hypertens* (Greenwich). 2012 Apr;14(4):265-6.

3   Intersalt Cooperative Research Group, "Intersalt: an international study of electrolyte excretion and blood pressure. Results for 24 hour urinary sodium and potassium excretion." *BMJ.* 1988 Jul 30; 297(6644): 319–328.

4   Leshem M, "Salt preference in adolescence is predicted by common prenatal and infantile mineralofluid loss." *Physiol Behav.* 1998 Feb 15;63(4):699-704.

5   http://www.watercure.com/ Accessed 11/06/2015.

6   Morris MJ, et al., "Salt craving: The psychobiology of pathogenic sodium intake." *Physiol Behav.* 2008 Aug 6; 94(5): 709–721.

7   Ahmed SH, "Is sugar as addictive as cocaine?" *Food and Addiction: A Comprehensive Handbook.* Eds. Brownell KD and Gold MS. Oxford 2012, p. 321–327.

8   Schiffman SS and Rother KI, "Sucralose, a synthetic organochlorine sweetener: overview of biological issues." *J Toxicol Environ Health B Crit Rev.* 2013;16(7):399–451.

9   http://drcarolyndean.com/magnesium_miracle/ Accessed 11/06/2015.

10 Schussler P, et al., "Ghrelin levels increase after pictures showing food." *Obesity* (Silver Spring). 2012 Jun;20(6):1212-7.

11 Greer SM, et al., "The impact of sleep deprivation on food desire in the human brain." *Nat Commun.* 2013;4:2259.

12 http://news.berkeley.edu/2013/08/06/poor-sleep-junk-food/ Accessed 11/06/2015.

Printed in the United States
By Bookmasters